Creative Writing

For The Mind, Body & Soul

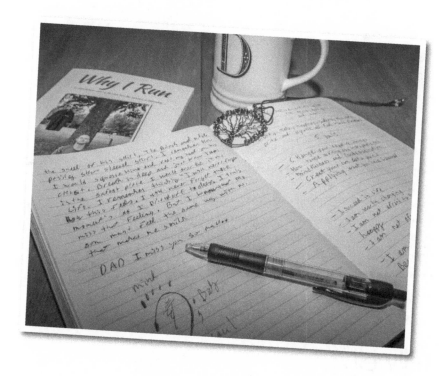

Darcy Patrick

Edited by Samantha Green
Cover Art by Dawn Hamilton

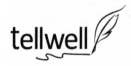

Tellwell Talent
www.tellwell.ca

ISBN
978-1-77370-470-8 (Paperback)

Contents

Foreword

I started therapy for depression in 2013. Soon after starting therapy, I began writing, which was part of my therapy itself. I learned to embrace writing and the power it gave me: I learned to write with honesty and love for my thoughts and emotions. This allowed me to become more open to using my new tools, and changing my way of thinking. I learned to prove my negative thoughts wrong using these tools, such as thought records and journal entries.

Over time, I learned to unleash the power of my mind by practicing mindfulness and writing out my experiences. I learned about guided meditation and started to create my own techniques. With help from my therapist, I created a safe place to go to in my mind when I felt a trigger in my life, which previously would have started a downward spiral in my mental state.

It was at this time that I wrote a book called "Why I Run: My story of how I won my life back from the darkness of depression". In this book I wrote about how I changed my life by learning to apply all the tools I was being taught to use in therapy, in hopes of helping other people. It was important for me to let others know that the way they felt, I felt too, letting them know they weren't alone and that if I could change, so could they.

"Why I Run" worked to say the least- in just one year, I sold over 2,000 books and helped many people with my message. I became a public speaker, doing talks all over Southern Ontario with the goal of breaking the stigma behind depression. Throughout this life change that I experienced, I had one thought on my mind at all the times: I wanted to make a difference in peoples' lives, and do everything I could to prevent deaths related to depression and mental illness.

Creative Writing for the Mind, Body & Soul is a very unique writing course. It will teach you to do thought records and journal entries. You will learn how to practice mindfulness, guided mediation, and to create your own safe place. But the most exciting thing you will take away from this experience is the freedom to learn all of this in your own way, at your own pace; there will be no right or wrong answers. There will be only you, with your thoughts, fantasies, and emotions. You will unlock the power of your mind, and you will learn to love life and set yourself free- in mind, body and soul.

Darcy Patrick

Course Outline

For this course, you will need a journal (which you can purchase from any book store), and a pen or a pencil. If you would like, you can also do this course on your tablet, laptop, or even your phone. Select the medium that you feel most comfortable using.

I first started writing using a program on my phone. I felt secure with a diary program at first because it allowed me privacy when I wrote. I eventually transitioned into writing in a journal, once I felt comfortable with what I was writing. I found that writing things in an actual journal, being one hundred percent open about my feelings, was part of my journey. We all have to feel comfortable in order for this program to work, and there are no right or wrong ways to do this. Write the way you feel most comfortable and free to express yourself.

In order to be successful at this program, you will also need an open mind and the willingness to change. By being open to this experience you will unlock the true power of your mind and go to places mentally that you've never dreamed of going. You will also learn to treat yourself with the love and kindness you deserve!

CREATIVE WRITING FOR THE MIND, BODY & SOUL WILL COVER THE FOLLOWING 5 GOALS:

1. Change your negative thinking.
   - Learn to notice and accept your negative thoughts and emotions by writing them down, learning that in doing so you free yourself from them.
   - Prove those negative thoughts wrong by using tools such as thought records and journal entries to conquer and organize them.
   - Learn to write with honesty, and in doing so realize that changing your life and thoughts is not out of reach. It is possible!

2. Learn to use writing as a therapeutic tool.
   - Learn to write out your secrets, your difficult thoughts, your emotions and how you feel about yourself. When you learn to do this, you are actually creating a safe place where there is no right or wrong, just your feelings.
   - Creating your own affirmations and learning that saying them and writing them every day will inspire you, build your self-confidence and cultivate a stronger you!

We are all entitled to our own feelings, and having a place where you can be free to express them is a wonderful gift to have.

3. Mindfulness and guided meditation
   - Learn to write a guided meditation.
   - Practice mindfulness in your writing.
   - Learn to use all 5 senses in your writing. This will inspire you and help you more easily reach a meditative state.

Through guided meditation you will unlock the true power of your mind, and celebrate it by creating your own meditations.

4. Create your own safe place
   - Using the tools from guided meditation and mindfulness, you will create your own safe place in your mind.

- Practice going to your safe place both as a writer and in daily life! Learn how it can become a place you can go to at any time, whether you feel overwhelmed or trapped (or just for fun!). This is a special place you create for yourself which is unique to you, and you can go there any time you need to.

5. Applying what you have learned
    - Reflect on what we have learned about writing and how it frees you!
    - Come up with your own ways to apply what you have learned in daily life and real life situations.
    - Use writing as a tool to practice acceptance of difficult thoughts and feelings, and in doing so learn to fight depression and anxiety.
    - Discover that using all these tools for yourself in your own ways will help to make your mind stronger, and will change your life.

Change Your Negative Thinking
Writing What You Feel

The power of writing your thoughts and emotions on paper is very therapeutic. It allows you to get your thoughts and emotions physically out of your body instead of letting them fester inside your mind. It also allows you to express yourself in a manner that you can relate to because the act of writing is a physical thing, so you will see what you have written and you will feel relief. You will be able to read over what you have written and see how you felt; the good, the bad and the ugly- it doesn't matter what the emotions are, you just write how you feel.

Once you start writing, you can go back and read old entries and feel good about how you dealt with situations in your life. This will reinforce the fact that you can deal with these situations because of what you have written in the past, and illustrate how you learned to overcome your problems.

Learning to write with honesty and love for yourself is the first step. Just writing out your emotions without being afraid and realizing it is okay to feel the way you feel is a great feeling.

Let's start with just a simple exercise by writing out the emotions we have about starting this creative writing course.

First, start with the date and a title. Place this anywhere you'd like on the page.

Example:

June 9/ 2017. My thoughts on starting "Creative Writing for the Mind, Body & Soul."

Now write what you feel, and remember to write with honesty. There are no rules, no guidelines. Just write, and do not be afraid of what you write as these are your thoughts and this is your time., Enjoy the freedom that you are being given to just write whatever you'd like. No one will get hurt.

I feel excited and overwhelmed at the same time. I have never been a good writer, and this is out of my comfort zone. I want to succeed and better my life. I feel proud that I am taking a big step here!

Once you are finished writing, read through what you have written and make sure it is what you really wanted to say. If you want to add to it feel free, all good writers proofread what they have written to make sure they have accurately captured what they want on paper.

Once you are done that, read through it again and see if you can pick out the emotions you are feeling. Are you happy because you are doing something to better your life? Nervous, because you have never written anything like this before? Bored, perhaps, because you have done this type of task before? It doesn't matter what you wrote, just as long as you acknowledge your emotions.

Example:

I feel excited and overwhelmed at the same time. I have never been a good writer, and this is out of my comfort zone. I want to succeed and better my life. I feel proud that I am taking a big step here!

Emotions: Excited, overwhelmed, uncomfortable, proud.

Learning to own/acknowledge your emotions is a hard thing because sometimes they are just so powerful that they consume you and you feel trapped by them. Learning to acknowledge them and write them down like we just did in the first exercise is the first step to learning how to deal with them.

We are rarely taught to deal with negative emotion in our lives; the positive ones are always easier to process. When we are happy, we smile and we feel good- if something is funny, we laugh. But what happens when a negative situation occurs in our lives? For some people, it is no big deal, they just acknowledge it and let it go without a second thought. For some of us, though, it is just not that easy. We have to learn to deal with these situations in a way that we feel comfortable, and doing this takes practice (and then more practice.) Over time we start to feel comfortable using our new tools and then we actually enjoy using them, because they start to feel good.

Let's Talk About Emotion: Introducing You To Journal Entries

Humiliation, pride, joy, love, hate, happiness, sadness, and guilt- these are the emotions that we all feel at sometime in our lives. Each and every one of us will experience these, it doesn't matter how old we are, if we are male or female, or what race or culture we come from; emotion is universal and we all feel it because we are all the same inside.

The next exercise will give you some practice writing about your emotions. You are to pick three emotions and write about them each day for 3 weeks. You can write about past events in your life where you felt a certain emotion, or you can write about things that happened to you that day.

The only rule to follow for these entries is that the last emotion you write about each time will always be a happy one. You will have to write about a happy time in your life, whether it's a fun time with a friend, something really funny that happened to you, or even a funny joke. But you will always end with a happy emotion!

Your exercises will look like this:

Date

Sept 12/2017

(*Emotion*) Humiliation

Today at work, after I posted the cleaning list, a senior staff member made fun of the list in front of the other staff members.

Body

This was humiliating to me because I was asked to post these cleaning duties as part of my job, so that the chores get spread out among all staff members on a weekly basis, so no one is having to do the same job all the time. This made me feel so small and childlike, like I was a joke in front of everyone in the store whom I am supposed to be the manager of.

(*Emotion*) Anger

I came home from work today and the sink was filled with dirty dishes

Body

When I came home from work today the sink was filled with dirty dishes. We have a dish washer and it never gets filled. Why can't other people fill the dish washer? Now I have to go into the dirty, cold water and take all the dishes out, and place them in the dish washer. This just boils my blood.

(*Emotion*) Happiness

Today I came home from work and went to the park.

Body

Today when I got home from work, it was very sunny out, so myself and my son went down to the park and played Frisbee together. It was such a nice way to end the day, laughing and running and playing together.

Doing these journal entries will build your confidence in acknowledging your emotions, and you will get used to writing about them and not feeling strange or uncomfortable about truly feeling them. Sometimes we feel guilty for feeling some emotions because they are negative, but you have to learn that every emotion lives in us, and having them is not bad and is not something to be ashamed of. Holding on to them and not letting them out or not letting them go is where the problems start. Over time you will just write your emotions without thinking, and you will feel comfortable and free to write as much as you'd like. If you get on a roll with this exercise, write every day if you can! Having emotions is not a bad thing and it just makes us human. Whether we like it or not we are all human and we all feel emotion.

Thought Records, Quick Thought Records, And So Much More

When you are depressed, you often have trained yourself to think in a negative manner. When something happens in your life that is bad and makes you feel uncomfortable, or emotional, you may think it has to be your fault or the world is against you and you can never win. These feelings control you and they dominate your thoughts, and in doing so they stop you from living your life.

When you are in this negative state of mind, you believe that you are one hundred percent correct in your thinking and that there is no way you could be wrong. You think this way because you feel that being in control and knowing that you are right will protect you from these things when they happen, but allowing these thoughts actually grows your depression. You are separating yourself from the outside world, internalizing your emotions, and not rationalizing them out - *"It is this way because I said so, and there is no way I am wrong!"*

When you think this way, you are using one-sided thinking. I like to say that the blinders go up and the world closes in, and you see only what you want to see. It is very hard and scary to acknowledge this because any other solution to your problem is just totally out of reach and absolutely wrong. The truth is that there are a number of different ways to look at things in our lives, you have to learn how! Just like riding a bike, playing a musical instrument, painting etc. We don't roll out of bed and become the greatest at everything we do in life, it takes practice. Before we know it though, we just ride that bike, we play that guitar, we just paint the picture. It is the same when we start to change our negative way of living. We have to learn to change our thoughts and how we react to emotion when it hits us.

In the last section, we practised writing out our emotions and three times a day for three days out of the week. Now we are going to learn to challenge these negative emotions in our lives and change our way of thinking to gain control of our lives. This is going to be exciting because we are going to take control in a positive manner. We are going to practice and then practice and practice some more, just like riding that bike. Over time it is going to feel natural, you will actually look forward to using these tools everyday.

Below is an excerpt from my book Why I Run explaining how I write thought records.

Thought records are a way of proving yourself wrong. You write down your thoughts at that time, acknowledging what is making your moods go a certain way, and then for each line you write you counter it with a real thought that proves that what you're thinking is actually wrong.

Below is the thought record I had after we tried installing my safe place for the first time.

Thought record:: I went to therapy

Situation::

I went to therapy and it was going well. We tried to create a safe place. I broke down crying and was just a complete mess.

Mood::: Scared 80%, Sad 100%, Distressed 100%

Thoughts::

I'm useless I will never get better. I'm better off dead.

I'm not useless. I passed level 2 training at work. I can do a thought record. I'm a good father and husband. I help people every day.

Why could I not do this? I feel I can never do anything right.

I do things right all the time. I do all the shipping and receiving at work. They trust me with that and I do it well. I'll be able to do create a safe place next time.

Mood:: relaxed 100%

This is how I do thought records. I learned about thought records from my therapist and from a book called Mind Over Mood by Dennis Greenberger, then I tweaked the technique a little and made it my own; you can do the same if you'd like, because there is no right or wrong way to do a thought record. This is a tool you can use any way you'd like, just as long as it works. Here is an example of how I write a thought record.

1. The title. I like to do the title of a thought record first, because it makes it easy to go back and find what I was having a problem with. It also helps to clarify what I was actually thinking at the time when I started to spiral or get upset over something. Here is a kind of fun title I will use to demonstrate a thought record:

Thought record title:: Moe going poop on a walk.

2. the situation (*or use a short form, as I do, and just write "SIT::"*). I write down what factually happened. I don't express any emotions here. I just write down what happened, plain and simple. Just the actual situation, nothing else. Here is an example of how this works in a thought record:

SIT:: I took my dog Moe for a walk. It was a sunny day, and we got to a corner when Moe went up to a tree and took a poop; I had no bag on me to pick up his mess.

3. The mood. Now I write down the moods I'm feeling at that time, how this situation made me feel, and how strong this feeling was. I use percentages, rating the mood's strength from 0 to 100.

For example, after I have described the situation above with Moe, I would write, "Moods::: Embarrassed 100%, Ashamed 100%"

The fourth step is the fun part: write down every thought that you have, and the emotions that triggered you in whatever situation you are in. This is the hardest part because you actually have to write down the truth! You have to be honest with yourself, otherwise the thought record will not work. I found this to be very difficult because I actually had to feel the emotions, not block them. I had to own up to what I was thinking when this situation was happening: no acting here, but 100% honesty.

It is hard work because we believe that what we were thinking when our emotions were triggered is the truth, and that our thoughts are right. Why wouldn't they be? We are always right in our thoughts and feelings!

Wrong!

When you are depressed, you have taught yourself bad habits and bad thoughts, and now you have to own up to them and prove yourself wrong. My therapist always told me try to think of it as if you are helping out a friend and they came to you with these thoughts.. You would help a friend if they came to you with a problem. People do it all the time, myself included. I will give my friends the best advice ever and not even think twice about it, but try doing it to yourself. Try to explain to a depressed man or woman that their thinking is wrong. Good luck! But here we go, we're going to do it. It takes practice, a lot of practice and a lot of repetition, thought record after thought record. I will talk about thought records in this book a lot because they are a huge tool in organizing your thoughts, and learning to use this tool is key.

Thought:::

I am ashamed of myself because Moe pooped on a tree, and I don't have a bag to clean it up. The owner of the house is on his front porch, watching, and I am so ashamed of myself for not having a bag.

Here is my counter thought:

I shouldn't be ashamed. It is a nice sunny day, I was in a hurry to get outside and forgot to bring a bag with me. There is no shame in what has happened here at all. I am human. I forget things.

Another negative thought:

This is horrible. This man is watching me and I don't have a bag. He knows I live around the corner, and now he will see me all the time and think of me as the guy who never cleans up his dog's poop! How will I ever walk down this street again? What a loser I am.

Counter thought:

I am not a loser, and I can just come back and pick up the poop later. I am not a bad man. All I did was leave some dog poop beside a tree. I can walk down the street anytime I like. Who cares if one day I didn't clean up poop right away? I'll come back.

It's as easy as that.

That is an example of a thought record, and one that is pretty straight-forward. Do you see how I countered my thoughts and made myself feel better, to see the situation for what it really was? I had to be honest with myself. I had to feel no shame in forgetting a little plastic bag. I had to accept that I am human and I make mistakes. Changing the way you think is not easy at all when you are depressed. You think you are always 100% correct, and that the situation you are in is 100% real, but it isn't, not at all, and only practising these thought records over and over again will change the way you think. I am telling you, kicking at the Darkness till it bleeds daylight is a constant fight.

Here is an overall breakdown of the structure of a thought record, so that you can follow along when creating your own.

-Title

-Situation (*Write with honesty and describe how you saw this event happen to you*)

-Moods/ Emotions (*how strong they are, using percentage as a rating system*)

-Thoughts that hit you right away (*Again, write with honesty and do not pull any punches- the truth and nothing but the truth*)

- Counter thoughts (*Now you can have fun thinking of different ways to view each thing you wrote*)

Write as many things down as you feel. Sometimes there are only a couple of thoughts to write down, other times there are way more. There are no rules to this. and sometimes a solution is just there right way.

-Moods after you have countered your negative thoughts. Be sure to use percentages again.

This is a standard thought record layout that should be practiced everyday, over and over again. You will bring your journal with you everywhere you go. My journal is always with me, never out of reach, whether I am at work or even out to dinner. I make no exceptions to the rule on this because proving my negative thoughts wrong is a lifelong journey for me and I enjoy doing it, and over time you will as well.

The assignment for this section is to write at least two thought records per day, everyday. You are by no means limited to only two a day, write more if you have to; in fact, I strongly suggest doing so. This is your chance to organize your thoughts and feelings.. Take the time to treat yourself with love and care, because that is what you are learning to do with these thought records – they are your thoughts and innermost emotions, so give them the time they deserve.

Quick Thought Records

Quick thought records are used when a situation happens in your life and you notice right away that it has upset you and know what the trigger is. Using this type of thought record can be the most rewarding because you are going after the thought right away and proving it wrong instantly. This makes you feel good about yourself and builds pride in the fact that you are progressing in your thought process. You have the ability to assess any situation, and you are now able to just write it out without any second guessing. Here is how they work.

(*Title*) Alex called and cancelled on a night out

(*Situation*)

My friend Alex and I have had plans for over a week to go out. He just called to tell me he can't go. He was in such a hurry that he didn't even give me an answer for why he is not going out with me. All he said was I will call you tomorrow.

(*Now write out your thoughts and then prove them wrong. Separate your counter thoughts with "//" and write out the alternative thought. See below.*)

Does he not like me any more? // No, don't be silly- he is a long-time friend.

Did I do something to piss him off in some way? // I haven't seen him since we made the plans a week ago. I couldn't have pissed him off.

No one ever likes hanging out with anymore, I must be the problem here. // No, Alex was in a hurry and didn't have time to talk, maybe he has a family crisis? His mother has been ill and maybe she isn't doing well and Alex had to go to be with her.

(*Now the solution to your problem*)

I will wait for him to call tomorrow and explain why he had to cancel. I can still go out, so maybe I will call another friend or go by myself? There is no reason why I should stay home on a Friday night.

As you can see, I wrote each thought out as they entered my mind. I countered each thought right away with a positive statement. In the past I would have not countered at all. I would have let my anger grow inside me, I would have cycled through the many reasons why Alex did not want to hang out with me, and I would have made it my fault by jumping to conclusions that were not real. I would have ended up feeling sorry for myself and just stayed home, letting this situation bring me down. Instead I used the quick thought record and came up with a solution to my problem.

Practice doing quick thought records everyday. They don't have to be long, they just have to be helpful. Sometimes you may only need to do one and sometimes you may need to do ten but sooner or later it will become natural and fun!

This part of the creative writing course is very important and is the basis for everything else we are going to work on.. Learn to love writing in your journal and do it everyday. Journaling can become an everyday event in your life. Writing can become your best friend. Start each day by writing in the morning. Whether it is planning out your daily events, or just writing how you feel in that moment, using the thought records, quick thought records, and journal entries is all part of bettering yourself and changing your thoughts.

Using Writing As A Therapeutic Tool

So far, we have learned to write out our emotions: the good, the bad, and the ugly. We also learned how we can prove our thoughts wrong by doing thought records and journal entries. We have learned to write with honesty and to do it daily when we need to. We feel comfortable writing and we use it to fight off downward spirals. Now we are going to use writing just for ourselves, and we are going to turn it into a type of therapy.

When you sit down and write, you are in a safe place. This is a place where you are free to write your feelings, your deepest thoughts and even your most intimate fantasies. We are all entitled to these things in life, there are no exceptions.

Writing allows you to bring your thoughts and fantasies to life! Celebrate them because they are no longer just in your head, but now they're on paper right in front of you (or on your computer screen, depending on how you wish to express yourself). The freedom that you unleash when you start writing with your heart and soul without second guessing is one of the most liberating and self-fulfilling things you can do for yourself.

Learning that this tool can heal difficult challenges in your life is a major bonus. You can write about your challenges, and how they affect you. Now is your time to let loose and finally say what you want to say. Talk about how you were hurt and how it changed you over time. When you write, you answer to no one. This is your time, so whatever you want to write is up to you! Nothing you write will ever hurt anyone! The only thing that can happen is that you will feel good about writing and freeing yourself from these challenges.

Freedom of expression is the gateway to happiness and self love. Taking the time to do something for you and you alone is not a selfish act, but an act of love and kindness. We all deserve to be happy, and we all like to be treated with love. Turn writing into a special place just for you, a place where you can do what you like. Take some time out of your day and dedicate it to writing for you and you alone. Write freely and with love, because you deserve to be happy.

Here are two examples of what writing freely and openly might look like, though it will be a different experience for everyone.

Grade school

When I was in grade school, I could not pronounce the letter "r" and even saying my name (Darcy) came out as "Docy." I hated it and was humiliated everyday when I was in class. It got to a point where I would not raise my hand to answer questions anymore because I would have to talk, and my classmates would make fun of me every day. Because I wouldn't talk in class, my teachers treated me differently, and eventually they sent me to special education classes because they thought I was stupid. I was not stupid. I knew the answers to the questions; I just didn't want to answer them. I also had a very hard time reading out loud because of the letter "r" and my classmates would always laugh at me. Even when I was in high school I had a hard time reading out loud.

I used to count the number of people there were in my classroom and then I would count the number of paragraphs there were in the book we were reading from. I would practice my paragraph before it was my turn to read out loud, and I would still screw it up. I remember there was a girl I liked in my English class and I had to read out loud, and I totally screw up and mispronounced the letter "r". I then started to stutter as well because I was so nervous. This girl looked at me and said "My god, you're so dumb..." and it destroyed me. I refused to read out loud in class again. When the teacher said it was my turn I would just say "No, I am not reading out loud ever again so don't ask me to." I hated that this happened to me, I hated that the whole time I was in school I was always a joke and looked at as being dumb. I hate that the girl in my class thought I was stupid. It has affected me my whole life. My self-esteem has always suffered because of that time in my life.

But it is all over now! Look at me: I have already written one book and I am a public speaker, I read out loud at every speaking event, I read out of the book **I** wrote! And if I miss pronounce the letter "r" I just smile and I think to myself, "Screw you grade school and high school and college. Look at me now, a published author, doing talks on depression and helping people everyday. I am the furthest thing from stupid!"

That was a bad experience in my life, and writing it out made me feel good. Ending it in a healthy way is even better because I looked at where I am now, and how wrong my thinking was back then, so I ended that chapter of my life in a positive way.

Below is a good experience I had while meditating beside my pond, and remembering that experience was very therapeutic.

Good Experience (Taken from my novel Why I Run)

This morning I took a little time to myself. I did yoga on my patio at water level beside my pond. I listened to my surroundings, my pond's waterfall, birds chirping as the sun rose, and I went through all my poses and held them all for two minutes. It was a full two hour routine.

It felt so good to be outside doing yoga, I had thought about it many times while downstairs in my basement office during the cold winter. Seeing the blue sky above me and the clouds floating by being surrounded by nature was just breathtaking.

It felt so good to take this time out for myself to treat myself to this wonderful experience. It is so important to just do simple things like yoga and feel the happiness which it brings. I am learning so much about life, and how important happiness is to live a healthy life. There are no life-threatening things happening to me, no matters in my life that have to be dealt with. I will live and enjoy life, be happy and learn everyday just what it means to be happy and learn there is nothing that needs to be done. My happiness is truly what matters. I look forward to the days that come. The many times I will sit and do my yoga beside my pond this spring and summer.

I hope my examples inspire you to write and make writing a therapeutic experience, so that you feel comfortable and free to write whatever you want to write! Expressing yourself is important and in doing so you set yourself free at the same time! Learn to use writing as a therapeutic tool.

Your exercise for this section will be to take time out of every day to write for yourself, and when you are finished, you are to end with a positive statement that frees you and inspires you, makes you feel good!

Affirmations

Affirmations are personal statements about ourselves which we want to believe. We will pick five affirmations that we want for ourselves, write them down, and we will explain why we picked them and the meanings they have to us. We will write them everyday at the end of any thought record or journal entry we do. Our affirmations will become our backbone and our source of pride because we will believe them one hundred percent. They will keep us strong and inspire us everyday. I would like to share my affirmations with you, and then you will come up with you own.

My Affirmations

When my therapist told me to make affirmations for myself, it was kind of funny because it made me think of this Saturday Night Live skit that I used to watch. The skit featured a guy sitting in a chair. His name was Stuart Smallie, and he would look into the mirror and say silly things about himself and people would laugh. The skit was very popular at the time, so I was kind of taken aback by what we were doing in this session.

It kind of felt like a joke to me, and I really didn't want to feel humiliated or embarrassed at therapy (or look like a fool like Stuart Smallie!) by saying anything silly. I was open to anything that could help me, and so far everything has worked, even though I initially didn't think it would.

I was told to come up with five affirmations that I believed in and write them down. These affirmations seemed silly at first, but they are actually my lifelong goals now. They help me all the time and I write them down in my journal every day. Sometimes I even say them out loud to remind me who I am. They help me get through tough days. Here are my affirmations. They are unique to me, and I will explain each one and why I have it.

1. I succeed in life.

This has been a major thorn in my side. In the past, I only looked at my failures and never my triumphs. Saying this affirmation made me think about the things I have succeeded at. The wording is so important here. There is no doubt in the phrase and to say it makes me feel good.

I succeed in life. Writing it and believing it and saying it out loud is so empowering. Thinking of just the things I have succeed at, it blows me away at times how I overlooked all the good and let the bad bring me down for so long. What a powerful thing writing and speaking something can be. When we were young we were taught a phrase that was so wrong: "Sticks and stones will break my bones, but names will never hurt me." What a lie! But it works both ways. Words can hurt, but they can help enormously, too. Saying things over and over and writing them over and over and believing those words works!

I succeed in life. So simple, but so powerful.

2. I am worth changing.

It breaks my heart when I say this one and write it, because for so long I felt that I wasn't worth changing. It has been such an uphill battle, learning and fighting, but this phrase is right! I am worth changing.

I am learning to love myself. I am learning to value myself. I am worth changing. I am worth the time and money. To invest in one's own self is the greatest investment of all. Change is a good thing and knowing that you are worth changing is the first step.

Many times I felt I was not worth the skin I was in, but not anymore. Now I know different. I am worth changing and everyone is worth changing.

Everyone deserves to be forgiven. I've got news for you: the most important thing is you need to forgive yourself. Realizing that you're worth changing is the first and foremost thing. I am worth changing!!

3. I deserve to be happy. I am not afraid to be happy!

"I deserve to be happy". What is that? For so long happiness was so far out of reach. Even emotion was at times out of reach. But I've got good news: everyone deserves to be happy. Whether it is playing with your son or sitting quietly on your back porch with your wife, not talking at all, just holding hands and loving each other. Happiness is something we all deserve in life. Some people need to learn that it is okay to feel happy. That's okay. What comes naturally to some doesn't to others and that's where the "I am not afraid to be happy" affirmation comes in.

I was so afraid to show emotion at all, never mind happiness, that anything was out of reach. I could act like I was happy. Hell, I was the best actor of all time. But not anymore. I am setting myself free and this phrase proves it to me. How strong is it?? Just say it with me and you'll see

I DESERVE TO BE HAPPY! I AM NOT AFRAID TO BE HAPPY!

It works. I know it does. I say it every day!

4. I am not afraid to be myself.

This one is scary.

I had lived for so long just trying to make other people happy. Everything I was about was making people happy. All I ever did was to make friends and make people like me. It was time for me to be myself and I was ready because this phrase says I am.

"I am not afraid to be myself."

I am not afraid is the key. Now I stick to it. I will say this in my head whenever I feel that I need to or when I am in a situation where I would normally bend and break, rather than be myself. I just say it and set myself free.

"I am not afraid to be myself" and if people don't like who I am then it doesn't matter, because not everyone is going to like me and now I can live with that. I can live with the fact that some of my friends may not like me and may not be my friends after all. I can live with the fact that I love who I am, and seeking approval for things I do is wrong and always has been. And guess what? "I deserve to be happy." "I am not afraid to be happy." "I am not afraid to be myself."

5. I am a strong and smart man and I will beat depression.

The best was saved for last. All through school, both grade school and high school, and then college, I was convinced I was stupid and less of a person than I really was.

My whole life I was searching for approval from others and never having any faith in myself. I had no self-esteem. But that is not true anymore

"I am a strong and smart man." I believe that. I have worked hard at everything I have ever tried. Sometimes I failed and sometimes I succeeded. That has made me both strong and smart, because now I know so much about myself from all the hard work and from never giving up.

I have chased so many of my dreams and I fell short, but in doing so I learned so much. I stood at the edge and I looked down and I turned my back and ran. I left that bridge that same day I held my son in my arms for the first time. I was strong enough to pick up a phone one day and call for help. I stopped beating myself up day after day, and I have worked hard as I always do at everything I try.

These are my affirmations! I say them every day, and I also end all my thought records and journal entries with them; repetition is always the key when using these tools. When I end my thought records and journal entries with my affirmations, it fills me with confidence and pride because what I wrote is something that matters and enforces the good work I have done. You can do the same; pick five for yourself and make them your own. Make them mean something, as I did ,so that they are unique to you. Let them build you up and let yourself feel proud when you say them. Let this exercise empower you.

Mindfulness Introduction

Mindfulness was taught to me in therapy as way to slow my life down, and to learn to relax and enjoy life. At that time in my life I had a very hard time doing anything for myself without feeling guilty or selfish. Even the smallest act of kindness I would show myself felt unnatural and strange.

My behaviors were backwards and need to be changed, so my therapist introduced me to mindfulness. We started with a simple act of going to a coffee shop before work to just sit and drink my coffee, and do nothing but enjoy some time alone to myself. It was so hard for me to do this. My thoughts where "I could be at work right now getting things done before the store opened", or "I could be using this time to catch up on all these repairs." So as I sat there and had these thoughts running through my mind, I did something that I like to do and I wrote. I countered my thoughts and I wrote them down.

I could be at work right now getting things done before the store opened.// Why should I do that? I don't get paid for coming in early.

I could catch up on all these repairs.// Why should I take my time before work and use it for something other than what I would like to do? I deserve to be happy, I deserve to do things I love. Work is not my life!

So I started to use this time before work to actually enjoy something for myself, and who knew that what I enjoyed the most was actually writing! So now I was actually in a hurry to get to the coffee shop so I could sit and write! I ended up writing eighty percent of "Why I Run" in that coffee shop! And I still can be found there almost every morning before work, just sitting and doing something I love. It was not an easy task at first but over time it became natural. Just like everything in life, we can accomplish great things with practice (and more practice!) and before long the unnatural becomes natural.

WHAT IS MINDFULNESS? / PRACTICING MINDFULNESS

Mindfulness is taking notice off all the things around you. Taking great care to notice each detail of what you are doing, what you hear, what you see, how things taste and how they feel. Paying attention to all the detail in your life. By doing this, you train yourself to stop the racing thoughts and centre in on the wonderful things that are surrounding you. You learn to take joy in doing simple things and you get lost in the moment. Before you know it, the stress that once controlled you will have completely disappeared.

Practicing mindfulness

When practicing mindfulness, we learn to treat ourselves with love and kindness and we take the time for our selves to get lost in the moment and actually see and hear things we never did before. We learn that it is okay to have guilt-free experiences, and we learn that life is for living and that learning to do so is a completely natural thing.

To start practicing mindfulness, we are going to do a homework assignment that was given to me when I started it myself. It is called "peeling the orange".

My homework assignment was to eat an orange every morning. I was to take an orange and sit at my kitchen table and place a napkin in front me. Next, I was to pick up the orange and roll it around in my hand, noticing everything about the orange: how it felt, if it was soft or if it was hard, determine whether its skin was it slick, lumpy, bumpy, give it a little squeeze, etc.. I was to then look at the orange and notice what the skin looked like, noticing the texture of the skin and all the little imperfections which made it perfect unto itself. How it was yellow in some places and light orange in other places and dark orange as well, paying attention to every change in shade. I was to take note that this orange was unique and still just an orange, even though nothing about it was perfect.

Then I was to peel this orange and as I did, I watched and paid attention to every detail of the action. The sound of the skin as it came off the orange. How I had to break through the skin with my thumbnail. How I would carefully place the skin on the napkin. What was happening to the fruit as I peeled off the skin and the juices were squirting out, covering my hands. I would suck the juices off my thumb and fingers and get a taste for what was going to come next. Just a little tease for what the orange is going to taste like.

Once the orange was peeled I would then break off pieces of the orange and eat it slowly. With each bite, I was to take in all the flavours, notice how each bite of this orange was always different and unique to itself, and in doing so I was once again reminded that nothing is perfect in life, and that even this orange I was eating was not perfect but its own version of perfection because of it's different tastes and textures. When I was finished I took great care to clean up the orange peels and throw them in the garbage.

Your assignment will be the same as above for the next week, but you are to do this exercise every day and then you are to write about. Write every detail and draw on all five senses when you write. Your "peeling the orange" assignment must make use of all five senses.

You can practice writing about your five senses by writing what you see all the time, and on the next page are examples for you to read through that will help you learn to take the time to practice mindfulness and aide in this assignment as well.

Examples of senses

Sight:

I think of wonderful colours created by a sunrise, the mixing of the sun with the clouds making unique shades of red, blue, pink, and purple. When I am on a morning run I will look to the sky to see just what is happening, and I will make a mental note and remember what I saw and use it in my writing.

When walking to work I take notice of people's front yards and get a good look at what is growing. Big wonderful bushes with different shades of green, how thick they are and how their leaves intertwine to make a solid bush. Blooming flowers just exploding before my eyes. How unique each one is, and how their colours are so vibrant and special. I save all these sights in my mind and in doing so I am practicing mindfulness.

I remember trips with my family when I was child and with my own family now. Waterfalls, nature paths, lakes, streams, fast flowing rivers. Fun times with friends. Sight is the building block and the most powerful thing when meditating for me. I build on top of an image and bring in the other senses as I go. I transport myself to that time or place. I will also make up a place as well that doesn't even exist and make it a wonderful place just for me. If you can imagine it, then you can make it happen in your head.

There are no rules here, no restrictions to what you can picture in your mind; you can go anywhere you'd like at any time. Total freedom of mind and body is what we are after. This why we are meditating to get to these places, leaving the outside world behind.

Sound:

Sound is soothing and relaxing, and bringing sound into a meditation can transport you to where you would like to be pretty fast. I sometimes use the sound of my backyard waterfall to wash away my problems after a hard day, or start the day with a fresh and clean slate. Even in the dead of winter I will use my backyard waterfall to transport me to a summer day beside my pond.

There are so many relaxing sounds in the world which can be brought into your meditation. A calm breeze blowing through trees creating a calm rustling sound.

The calming sound of waves whooshing onto the shore of a beach. Birds chirping in the morning, toads calling to their friends. Sound is so powerful and repetitive sounds work best as they distract you from the outside world while creating an almost hypnotizing feeling.

Sometimes just hearing certain sounds can trigger memories. The sound of a dog catching a Frisbee – for example – brings me to a special time in my life where I would play Frisbee with my dog at a park close to my house. Just thinking about the sound now brings back an image I haven't seen in five years.

Use your imagination! If you are picturing a walk in the woods then try to hear the birds chirping, sticks snapping under your feet, breeze blowing the leaves in the trees. The sound of a creek gently running in the background, a squirrel climbing a tree. Capture all the sounds you may hear in those woods. Whatever the moment you are wishing to create, add whatever sounds go along with it, This is very simple but very effective for the overall exercise.

Smell

Smell can transport you to any place in a matter of seconds; even just a faint smell of something can trigger memories in our mind. Smell is so powerful and using it is so important. There are certain smells that just ignite our brains, bring goose bumps to our skin and make our hair stand on end at the back of our necks, even trigger memories of people who have passed away. The smell of your grandmother's perfume will bring back great memories of her, or maybe the smell of a pipe being smoked would trigger a mental picture of your grandfather sitting smoking his pipe after dinner.

Coffee percolating always makes me feel calm and relaxed. There are so many different smells you can describe and tie in with what you are seeing and hearing. Walking in the woods, bring the smell of wet, damp wood. Walking past a garden- the smells of roses, lavender, and honeysuckle blooming. If you're sitting on the beach, maybe you imagine the smell of wet sand or the faint smell of seaweed drying in the sun. A campfire burning as you sit with your family or friends roasting marshmallows. If you are on farm use farm smells, on a fishing trip sitting on a bank of a river then think of the smells you might come into contact with. Write down scents and build a list if you need help, A list of scents and where they come from will be helpful for you to draw on, if you're having difficulty thinking of how to tie them in to your setting.

If there is no smell to associate with your place then no problem, just leave it out and keep building. Again this is your meditation and you can make it anyway you would like it.

Touch(feeling)

Touch/feel is a big sense to draw on as it is so many different things. Touching something with your hands and feeling the various textures like soft, hard, slippery, wet, prickly, slimy, and so on. I like to practice enjoying the sense of touch when I am running. I will pull a leaf from a tree and rub it between my fingers and thumb, feeling it's texture and the veins that run through the leaf. Is it soft or waxy? Fuzzy on the underside? Or is it slick and slippery? I remember all these different textures and use them in my writing. When I am eating an orange, I will run my hand over its skin and feel the bumps and lumps before ripping it open to eat.

The tactile feeling part of the touch is the most exciting because it is what your body is literally feeling. For example, the sun warming your skin on a hot summer day while you are walking on a beach. The breeze cooling you off when you get out of a stream you were swimming in. The shock you get when diving into a cold lake up north at a cottage you are staying at in the middle of nowhere. Touch/feeling are strong senses and they have to be included in your meditation. Practice them by just enjoying your surroundings.

Taste

Finally, we are going to focus on taste, one of the most powerful senses. The explosive taste of an orange, a fresh ripe peach, a sour apple and grapes freshly picked from the vein are all things that make my mouth water just imagining them. Remember eating the best dinner you've ever had and biting into it; feeling the textures on your tongue, each movement of your mouth releasing new flavours. So many possibilities are there, you just have to draw on them.

One time I was in Montana on business, and I was treated to many a good meal. One stands out the most for me though: a bison steak I ordered at a restaurant I would have never been able to afford to eat at if not for the trip I was on.

I like my meat rare and I had never had bison before, so I was very excited when it came. Fresh vegetables grilled to perfection with grill markings seared on them accompanied the steak, including broccoli, red and green peppers and (my all time favourite) asparagus. The bison was the greatest thing on the plate, with just the right amount of red for me. I sliced into it with my sharp steak knife with a strong wooden handle, and it sliced the meat like butter. The meat was so tender and had zero fat, a perfect cut just for me. I put the small slice I had already cut into my mouth, and the taste was out of this world! The meat just melted and I barley had to chew. I could taste just a little bit of seared meat followed by a little bit of pepper they used for flavor. I followed it up with a bite of the grilled asparagus and then washed it all down with a swig of beer that was brewed locally, a dark amber ale with a very wheat after taste and a honey overtone.

This meal was outstanding and is burnt into my mind forever, mainly because of those flavours. The thought of those tastes alone transports me back to that dinner and the friends who were there, the laughter, and the music that was playing. The whole experience just comes back to life when I remember those flavours- taste is a powerful sense.

Use all five of the senses I just wrote about to help you in your writing, and once you start thinking in detail and really enjoying that detail, you are practicing mindfulness!

For the next week you are to wake up in the morning and you are to peel the orange and you are to take notice of everything that you experience and then write about it! Have fun and write just what is in you mind including what you see, touch, hear, smell and taste. Write with honesty and love, getting lost in the moment and exploring just how much of this experience you can savour!

Mindfulness is about getting lost in the detail and taking notice of the small things, so the more detail, the greater the experience. Enjoy this exercise make it our own and before you know it you will actually start enjoying this time to yourself. You may even find that your day will not feel right without eating that orange in the morning.

I would like to share a short excerpt from my book Why I Run where I used mindfulness to enhance my experience while I was running and also to relax me.

Thought record:

My run

This morning on my run, I took the time to lose myself and look at the beauty all around.

Moods:

Happy 100% Relaxed 90%

I looked at all the beautiful trees and their wonderful shapes and vibrant colours. The light greens, the dark greens, the reds, the browns and how alive they were. How different and unique each tree is: the shapes of their trunks and the flowers on the flowering trees. The bright pink and red colours of a cherry tree in the spring. The beautiful white snowball bushes as well. The wonderful smell of blooming lilacs and lavender.

I got a little selfish and pictured myself in one of these vibrant trees and how it must feel to be inside one bursting with life after a long winter and the exhilaration of flowering. It was fantastic. I also pulled a leaf off a tree and ran it between my fingers feeling its veins and its unique texture

I also ran past bushes and ran my hand over top of the new growth and felt the energy each bush had.

I looked up at the clouds and saw the beauty in the sunrise and marvelled at the colours that the sun and clouds were making together: the reds, the pinks, and the blue sky framing it all. It was just breathtaking.

I had a great 12 km run, and when I finished, I walked for 1 km and just breathed deeply and relaxed. I was amazed at how good I felt. 12 km and it felt like I had not even run at all.

This is a good thought record- who says they all have to be bad!

Guided Meditation

Guided meditation, to me, is a wonderful way to deal with the outside world. When I say this, I mean what the outside world brings to my life: stress from work, stress from family, stress from finances, worry, anxiety, guilt- I hope I didn't miss anything. Being able to take myself out of this crazy world and into a place that is calm and peaceful is a huge thing. I never thought that it would be such a major part of my life when I started, but now my days don't seem right without starting off with meditation.

Just taking the time for myself and starting the day calm and relaxed is a simple thing. Starting with a blank slate and an open mind makes the normal stress in life seem not so big or impossible to deal with. When my mind is clear and calm, my thought patterns are healthy and I am able to find solutions to problems instead of getting overwhelmed. Calm and level thinking is a major tool in living a happy life, loving who you are, and remembering that nothing in life is urgent or life threatening. When stresses come up (and they always do), I take the time to calm myself by meditating for even five minutes and I come out with a different outlook and a better frame of mind. Whatever was on my mind and stressing me out before meditating just doesn't have any power over me anymore.

Being calm and relaxed allows me to actually not act on emotion or react in an emotional way to situations which arise. I alone control my moods and being in a calm place allows me to use my tools I was taught to use in therapy, and change my negative thought patterns. Guided meditation is the key to using my tools and a major part of starting and maintaining a good day filled with happiness and positive thinking.

Learning to relax and calm yourself is the first step in learning to write a guided meditation and to practice it as well.

Learning to relax

Learning to start a meditation is no easy task. I still fight to empty my mind and push the outside world away as it is not easy to just turn off. But my secret is I don't turn off, I just redirect my over active thoughts to what I am trying accomplish. I do this by first finding a peaceful place. That can be anywhere you like, a park bench, in your bedroom on your bed, your living room floor or sofa, really anywhere you feel at peace. I have meditated sitting on a chair in the middle of a busy downtown street in front of my favourite coffee shop. Anywhere you feel comfortable is the right place to be.

Making sure I am 100% comfortable in the position I am sitting in is very important as well. Sometimes I am sitting cross legged in front of my pond and sometimes I am just sitting straight up in a chair, my feet on the floor and hands on my knees. Whichever way you sit, the main thing is that you feel comfortable in order to relax and calm yourself. If I am not comfortable I can never just relax, because my mind will be focused on how I need to change my position I am sitting in, and not on relaxing.

Now I breathe deep with a long inhale through my nose and I make sure I feel my chest lift, I feel the breath right to the end of my inhale and until I am full of air. I let out the air, and I exhale through my mouth. I direct my full attention to my breathing making sure I am 100% just paying attention to my chest rising and then falling on the exhale. Just paying attention to this and this alone will relax you, taking your mind off the outside world and all of its nonsense.

Just breathing deep and paying attention to your breathing is something we really never do throughout the day and breathing is what gives us life. It is also a dead giveaway for when stress hits us. Your breathing can speed up or become shallow, even have you gasping for air hyperventilating. Such a simple thing, to pay attention to our breathing. Deep, slow breaths, feeling your lungs expand and contract. Just breathe and think of nothing but that and that alone. Once I am totally relaxed and calm I let my mind go, and it goes in different directions- I let it go and I bring it back with concentrating on my breathing once again, and I will do this over and over again till my mind is finished bouncing from place to place.

Letting your mind bounce around once you are relaxed and bringing it back by concentrating on your breathing is practicing control over your thoughts, and is a form of meditation in itself. I will just sit and control my breathing and my mind for a whole meditation session. This breathing exercise is a very relaxing and calming thing to do, and you may have to do it a lot before you even bring in an image or any senses. This is the building block to guided meditation and must be practiced over and over again. The good news is it is good for you and you can do it anywhere, because breathing is what we do to live and just paying attention to it is natural and healthy. Learning to let go of your thoughts is no easy task but learning to bring your mind back from theses thoughts is essential.

When I am relaxing I like to do a simple exercise; I will breath deep, paying attention to my long inhale and exhale, I will then let my mind wander off to one thing and I will only allow this one thing in my mind. I will then bring my attention back to my breathing, and I will count to ten in my head as I breathe inward. On the exhale, I will only pay attention to the breath being pushed out. I will repeat this two times and then I will relax and let my mind wander again. I will bring myself back from where my mind wandered by counting to ten again on my inhale, and again only concentrate on pushing the air out on the exhale. I will practice this exercise throughout the day, before a run after a run, while having a coffee, on lunch break, while on a walk or just sitting by my pond.

When a stressful situation arrives at work I will close my office door and I will practice this exercise, letting the stress and the situation disappear and focus-ing on just my breathing. If you are feeling anxious and your body is reacting and show signs of being overwhelmed, do the breathing exercise you've just learned. Once you can do this then using you mind to create a guided medita-tion is just a step away.

We are going to learn to create our own guided meditations. We are going to use all the things that we have learned so far in this creative writing class to create our own special places. These will be places we can go to in our minds when we feel we need to, or when we just want to feel good and treat ourselves with love.

We will write with honesty and we will indulge in our own fantasies. We will allow ourselves to create a place just for us to go to and we will write it all down. We will draw on all of our senses as we write, we will transport ourselves there on paper and we will then burn that experience into our minds. Once we write it out it will become a memory and something that we can go back to in our minds when we want, and even add more detail when we go there to enhance our experiences.

Because of all the hard work we did doing thought records and learning to prove our negative thoughts wrong, we are now able to write with honesty and love. Not only that but we now know when situations hit us we can use mindfulness and meditation to help us get through them, and also build a meditation for each problem that arises in our lives.

Before we start, I would like to share a guided meditation I wrote where I expanded the "peeling of the orange" exercise to a wonderful place I like to go to.

The Orange

This morning my mind was racing, worries and stress soon crept in, feelings of being trapped and that nothing in my life will ever change played on my mind. I acknowledged my feelings and what was happening to me, I began to slow my thoughts down by closing my eyes and taking deep breaths and only paying attention to my breathing.

As I sat cross legged on my blue yoga mat, I just breathed deep and slow. I closed my eyes and pictured my tree standing before me, my safe place, my old friend. I walked over to my tree and ran my hand over its grainy bark feeling its nooks and crannies. I then stepped inside my tree I sat cross legged in its trunk levitating in the centre of it. I began to breathe in through its leaves and out through its roots, just making oxygen and paying attention to how my breath was flowing with its circulatory system. My breathing became one with the tree, with everything flowing together in through the leaves and out through the roots and back again. (Take the time now to go to the tree and enjoy the peace and calm of just being a tree and only enjoying your breathing. In through the leaves, and out through the roots.)

Once completely relaxed, picture yourself driving a red Ferrari (choose any car you dream of driving) through the rolling hills of an orange plantation in Florida. You come across a huge plantation that is filled with trees, large, old, vibrant trees stretching as far as your eyes could see. These trees are covered with ripe oranges. The sight is mind blowing, the green trees and the oranges highlighting the green background. You pull over the car at the side of the road just on the gravel shoulder. You get out of your car and stand there with amazement at the beauty before you. (close your eyes now and picture this image)

Before you are rows and rows full of orange trees stretching so far you cannot see the end of them. You walk across the street and stand at the edge of the plantation and a gentle breeze blows by, and the smell of fresh oranges ignites your senses (feel the breeze and imagine the smell). You walk into the plantation and say to yourself "I am going to eat one of these oranges." You bend down and take your shoes and socks off, and leave them at the edge of where the freshly groomed grass leading to the plantation starts. As you walk forward you let the grass massage your feet with every step you take.(Take the time now to walk in that grass, feel it.) You approached a fabulous mature tree, its limbs are huge and it has a wonderful shape to it. All of its limbs and branches create an intricate umbrella above you, shading you from the hot sun. You looked up and see the perfect orange, round and so vibrant, filled with juice and ready to burst at any moment. You reach up and have to stretch every muscle in your body to reach this orange and pluck it from its branch. The orange is the size of a soft ball and it is heavy ,ripe and ready to eat. (Picture this orange and imagine its weight as you hold it in you hand.)

You walk away from the tree with your prize, and you see an old fashioned hand pump off to your right. You take the heavy, swollen orange over to the rusty pump and begin to pump up and down on it, before you know it the pump is bursting out fresh cold water from the depths of it' well. (Picture the cold water rushing out and the feeling you have as it hits your hands.) You hold the orange in your left hand and pump the water over it with the right, washing the orange clean. Through the corner of your eye, off to the left you see a small round wooden table, it is only about one foot tall and about twelve inches around and there is a wood bowl sitting on. The bowl is about half way filled with orange peels, and there is a white cotton towel there as well for drying your hands off afterwards. You walk over and sit cross legged beside this table.(Picture the table now, try and see the detail as you walk over to it.) You take the ripe orange and take a bite out of the bottom of it. You pull the centre of the peel out with your teeth. The juice covers your face and the taste is out of this world, like no orange you have ever tasted; tangy and sweet at the same time. So fresh, your taste buds are put into overdrive.

You place the centre of the orange peel in the wooden bowl, and you begin to peel the orange with care. You dig your thumb in between the peel and the flesh of the orange and pull it back. (Imagine what is happening now. What sounds do you here as the peel is pulled away from the flesh of the fruit?) With each piece of orange peel you remove, your hands are drenched with its juices. You suck the juices off your thumb as you place the peels in the bowl.

Once the orange is peeled, break it in half and place one half on the table and the other half you will carefully peel each layer off and eat. The pieces of the orange melt in your mouth, each one sweeter than the one before. (Imagine the taste explosion with every bite you take, how each piece is an experience.) You finish the first half and move on to the second.

The second half you just pick up and take a big bite, and the orange explodes in your mouth, all over your face. The juices are running down your face and neck but you don't care, you just take another bite and enjoy this moment fully; the tastes, the sights, the smells and the sounds of this wonderful experience. After you're finished, you take the white towel and clean yourself up. You walk over to the hand pump and you wash your face off with the cold well water. You slowly walk over to where your shoes and socks are at the edge of where the gravel meets the grass. You slowly put your socks and shoes on. Before you leave, you take one more long look at this wonderful plantation. (Imagine what this place looks like, try to burn it into your mind and see, hear, smell everything.) You get back in your red Ferrari and drive away.

Now go back to the tree and breath deep and long once again, just taking air in through your leaves and out through your roots. When you are ready, step out of the tree and walk around it and give it a hug. Open your eyes and you are calm and happy, free from stress and feeling strong and proud!

The power of my mind blows me away at times. The times that I have spent stewing and worrying and sinking deep into a depressed state was a waste of my mind power. But then learn to create such a wonderful and vibrant place in my mind truly shows the power that each and every one of us has over our thoughts.

Sometimes I think that people like me who are blessed with an overactive mind just need a way to put that power to good use, and learn how to focus and draw on the good and not the bad in life. I say blessed with an overactive mind now, but before I thought I was cursed and only saw the bad in life. But to do a meditation like we just did is proof that our minds are capable of doing so many things in life, that just learning to focus and most of all practice ,practice, practice is the most important factor when learning new things and truly being happy.

Creating Your Own Guided Meditation

Step 1: Notice Your Mood

Creating your own guided meditation is such a fun and personal thing to do. I like to sit down and notice my mood at the time. Whether it is happy, sad, anxious, it doesn't matter: I sit and I think "Where do I wish go right now? What can I do for myself at this moment? Do I need to distract myself from a problem I am having, or do I just want to have fun and create the richest experience I can have?" Because you can have it both ways!

Step 2: Make Up A Place and Give it a Title

Now don't be afraid to go anywhere you want to, do anything you like – we are entitled to our own fantasies and our own dreams, your only boundary is your imagination! Give it a title so once you are finished writing it, you will always remember it, and you can go there anytime you'd like.

Here are some titles I have used in the past.
- Down on the dock
- The cabin in the woods
- Flying the clouds

- High on the mountain side

Just writing out each of those titles bring back memories from each one I wrote and they are now burnt into my mind.

Step 3: Relax and Write About It

This is the exciting part and the part I love the most because you now write out how you are going to relax. Simply breathe deep like we practice at the beginning of this section, and write about it at the same time.

Example:

I sit in my chair in my living room and I let myself sink into this chair I just relaxed and concentrated on my breathing and only my breathing. Feeling each breath from the beginning of the inhale and then out as I exhaled only paying attention to my breath.

(Now close your eyes and just take one minute to do this we are now connecting our mind and body together. We will write as we do this burning it into our mind and living it at the same time.)

Step 4: Writing About Our Place

Now write about the place you wish to go to, take your time to make it just as you want it to be and use as much detail as you can. (*Draw upon the exercise we wrote about when practicing mindfulness.*)

- Sight
- Sound
- Smell
- Touch
- Taste.

When you write after each detail, take the time to stop and close you eyes, and breath deeply. Bring yourself to picture what you wrote about, see it, hear it, smell it and taste it, feel it. Take your time and get lost in the detail both as you write and as you close your eyes and bring yourself there.

Sometimes I will write an entire paragraph and then sit and close my eyes and bring myself there, other times I will just write one description and just bring myself to that point and stay there for a while. There is no rush when writing a guided meditation, this is your time and you can write for as long as you'd like, and you can stop as many times as you like. Bring yourself to the place you are writing about, free your mind and enjoy your time there..

Step 5: Finish Off Your Meditation

When you are finished your guided meditation, write about it. How do you feel afterwards? Has your mood changed? What are your emotions? What did you like most about your meditation? Feel free to write exactly what is on your mind. Be proud and celebrate it.

Example:

After this meditation, I feel confident and relaxed. I love that I was able to bring myself to this place and I was able to experience everything like I was actually there! This is a memory I will keep in my mind forever! I can't wait to create my next guided meditation and I wonder where I will go tomorrow!

You just did an amazing thing by connecting your mind, body and soul through writing. Now the fun part is that you can now go to this place you just wrote about anytime you'd like and be free in your thoughts.

Sometimes when I am at work and the stress gets to me I will close my eyes and I will think about one of my meditations, and it will bring a smile to my face as I remember how I felt and the stress just disappears. I think about "The Orange" or "The Mountain Top." I remember that I have these great places and I remember that I went there, and most of all I remember just how powerful my mind is and that I control my moods and my emotions!

You don't have to write a new meditation every day, you can do them once a week. After writing it, go to that place every day for a week and then write a new one. Create favourites and learn to love them. Use them when you need to. Have one for releasing stress, have one for just being happy, have one for when you have nothing to do and you just want to sit somewhere and be at peace. There are no boundaries and no rules; just you and your mind!

Creating A Safe Place

A safe place is somewhere you can go to in your mind to escape the outside world, calm yourself and help stop you from being triggered into a downward spiral. This is different from guided meditation which we just learned about. It is different because this will be a place which will always be the same every time. You will learn to bring yourself there whenever you'd like to. The idea behind it is that you will ingrain the details in your mind in such a way that you will make it a completely personal experience. You will be able to bring yourself there quickly and with very little effort..

You will use all the tools which you put into practice when writing out your guided meditations. You will create a safe place just for you. Before we get started, I would like to share how I found my safe place, and then we will learn to create your own safe place. A place to have and love and go to when you feel the need to. But even better than that, a place where you can go and feel good about yourself and your accomplishments, because having a special place that is unique and just for you is a great accomplishment unto itself.

The following is an except from Why I Run, detailing how I found my own safe place.

Journal entry:

I need to talk to my therapist about why I can't let go of my emotions why I just can't be free from my thoughts. How there are always things on my mind. I never truly relax and just let go.

I am afraid when I do I'll just cry and cry and cry, and just explode with emotion. I have already done that when I wasn't even close to being completely relaxed? What's going to happen to me when I truly let go and let my emotions free after all these years? I am scared and terrified of that moment. I need to feel. I need to be free. I need to let go. I need to be me!! I need to go to this safe place and just let whatever happens happen.

What will happen? I am scared.

I was still spiralling and my therapist wanted to install a safe place that I could go to in my head, like a kind of meditation, to calm me down and make me stable again. Somewhere I could just be at peace.

Now the struggle started. I was so nervous about it I could not relax at all. I was convinced that it was just not going to happen. I could never create a safe place.

It was up to me to find my safe place, so I started.

Attempt #1

I pictured myself walking Moe my dog who I have recently put sleep to the park, us playing Frisbee .The sun was shining and there were pine trees lining the right side of the park and I could smell the morning dew and Moe was running and catching the Frisbee. I could feel the grimy dog saliva on my hand from throwing the Frisbee. I could hear Moe's teeth bite down and catch it as I threw it.

But picturing that didn't work. I could not go there. I could not relax and really I wasn't over Moe at all. The experience was a total disaster. I just broke down and was a mess. I was failing at another thing in life: I was not able to install a safe place and I had never come to grips with putting my dog to sleep....

So it was back to the drawing board for round two at the safe place...

Attempt #2

This time I was at the beach sitting on a beach chair and the sun was shining. It was hot. I was having a beer and the water was just washing up on the shore, nice and calm. My son Dylan was swimming and my wife Sherri was beside me. It was great my therapist was able to bring me there without a problem at all. But the last time I was at the beach was when I had just started therapy and I had a major break down and I ended up just thinking about that day and again I broke down and was a mess once again. I was a failure all over again.

Here is the Journal entry from that time at the beach when I actually broke down.

Journal entry:

At the beach

I hate my life. I'm trying to get better but wife Sherri is so angry and hates me for what I'm going through. What's the use anyway? I'm just going to keep living the way I'm living, unhappy and acting the whole time. So I don't hurt her and Dylan.

That day at the beach I fell apart in front of Sherri, tears and everything. She saw me at the worst.

I was going to break for real. I told her that sometimes I wish I was gone. I wish I would disappear. I told her that I'm not happy, that I have been acting for years and that I'm going crazy. I just fell apart. I was crying and shaking and I just spiraled down. What a way to spend our last days of vacation.

Attempt #3

So now it was time again to try something new. But my therapist just wanted to work on relaxation in general and so she introduced me to the tree meditation, which is one of my favourite things to do. I sit and breathe deep and just feel how my body is sitting and just notice everything that is around me. I close my eyes and just breathe deeply. She asks me what kind of tree I see before me. I tell her I see a large brown maple tree. I walk toward this tree and I magically just step into it and just breathe, breathe deeply. I slowly bring the air in through the leaves and push it down through my trunk and out into the ground through my roots and then in through my roots and out through my leaves. I just imagine I can feel the wind blowing me from side to side and I let my body move freely as this tree, just feeling relaxed and peaceful. She asks me what I am feeling, what emotions are flowing through me and I tell her and she just says go with that feeling and enjoy it for as long as you like. Then when you are feeling just right take a deep breath and step out of the tree and open your eyes slowly and stay in that emotion you were feeling. I open my eyes and step out and I am relaxed and at peace and holy smokes I feel so good.

Guess what? I found my safe place and it was fantastic!

I have grown the tree meditation into a beautiful, safe place. I go there all the time. It is so peaceful and I don't cry. I feel free and I can do whatever I like and I just step into a tree.

The tree is a perfectly safe place. When I need to go there, I walk around the tree and run my hand over its bark, feeling its roughness and its nooks and crannies, and kind of say "Hi" to this tree. I imagine that I have this gift and I just slowly walk into this tree and I feel its whole circulatory system and as I breathe I take the air in through the leaves and out through the roots. I feel the sap coursing through my limbs and I imagine the wind blowing my leaves around. I just feel everything the tree feels, like birds landing on me and even building nests and having baby birds living on me. I stay in the tree till I feel I have stayed long enough and whatever caused me to be stressed out has left my mind. The outside world can't touch me here. I am free from everything in the tree and that is so, so special.

When I walk out, I thank the tree and I give it a nice pat and once again rub my hand along its trunk to feel its bark and roughness. I walk away relaxed and complete and I take the tree's strength with me as I leave my special safe place.

I had over analyzed the safe place until I was terrified of it and I had all these expectations and worries about what a safe place was. A safe place is just that, a safe place, end of story. No over thinking and I can cry, I can feel whatever I want to because it's my safe place!

Thank you, Mastora, for my safe place.

Step 1: The Name

The first thing you need to do to create this safe place is to write down some places you might have in mind, take your time and write freely. You can choose many things, for example: a place in time that you felt good in, an activity that you enjoy doing, a good memory you may have from the past, or time spent with a friend.

Here are some additional examples:

- On the beach
- Ice skating
- Swimming in a lake or pool
- Flying like a bird
- A bike ride with a friend
- Exercising, Running, walking, playing a sport ect.

Once you have picked from your list, name it! Make it yours and yours alone.

Step 2: Use Your Senses

Bringing in the senses just like we did when writing out a guided meditation, think about the main things you want to draw on from this place.

Example:

riding my bike.

Sight

- What does the bike look like? Is it old or new?
- What colour is it? (don't be afraid to make it any colour you would like)
- What do you see while you are riding?
- Where are you riding to? Write about it.

Describe everything you see in great detail.

Sound

What do you hear?

- Is the bike noise?
- Birds chirping .

Feel

- Can you feel the wind as you ride?

- Is the road bumpy?
- What do the handle grips feel like?
- Is it hard or easy to pedal?
- Does it steer easily?

Smell

- Describe any scent in the air
- Someone barbecuing?
- The smells after a fresh rain.

Taste

- Do you have a drink holder? What type of drink do you have on your bike?
- Is your mouth dry from the wind as you ride?

Using your five senses, you can bring your safe place alive. The more detail, the better, and it will be easier for you reach this safe place.

Step 3: Making It Real

Write your safe place out and as you write it down, take the time to completely go there. Start with relaxing and breathing deeply like when we are doing a guided meditation. When you are relaxed, write out your title and just think about it for a while. Put yourself there mentally and picture it as if it were a real place.

When you have this picture in your mind, write out how you would like it to start. When you are finished writing, stop and go over what you wrote three times and then close your eyes. Picture yourself going there.

Once you are there, write the body of your safe place using the details you wrote out in step two as much as you can. Pay attention to how you are feeling emotionally as you do this and notice how your body is relaxed and free of stress. As you write, concrete on the good, happy feelings you are having as you create this safe place. Don't rush through this stage of writing and take as many breaks as you'd like.

Once you have the body written, start reading from the top of the page and make sure that as you read you are going there and seeing and feeling everything you have written. Once you have done this, write out how you would like it to end. As you write this out, again, pay attention to your emotions and notice how free and happy you are as you write your ending.

Once you are finished this exercise read it again over again and make sure that this is your safe place and you are comfortable in it. Love your safe place and think about it as you finish up reading it.

Step 4: Putting It In To Practice

Now that you have your safe place written out and you have read it over and over again, you will now put it into practice. Each morning when you wake up, you will go somewhere quiet and open you journal. Breath deeply and relax yourself, then you will read through your safe place from beginning to end, taking your time to really go there in mind and body. Once you are done you will close the book and once again go there in mind and body, this time noticing all your emotions and how your body feels while there. Once you are finished, go about your day as you normally would, but keep your safe place on your mind; even just saying the title every once in awhile will help to keep you calm and centred.

At lunch time you will start your lunch by closing your eyes and going to your safe place, this will only take you maybe 2 or 3 minutes to do, then eat your lunch and enjoy it. Once you are finished eating, go to your safe place again.

Have you ever heard the saying "whistle while you work?" For the afternoon while you work, just in the back of your mind, think about your safe place as you go about your day. Notice how you can carry the good emotions with you that accompany your safe place and notice how you can be completely relaxed as you go through your second half of the day Realize just how wonderful having a safe place can be.

At the end of your day, before you go to bed, reread your journal entry and allow your mind to travel to that safe space again. Make sure that you are allowing yourself to commit to this exercise one hundred percent, and when you are done you can put the book down and end your night.

You are to do this exercise every day for a week and enjoy the time you spend doing it. Sooner or later this safe place will become second nature to you, and will be an automatic and natural response to stress.

Step 5: Using Your Safe Place

Now that you have your safe place and you are able to go to it with ease and without struggling, you can start applying it!

I use my safe place when I feel I am getting overwhelmed, like I really can't control my emotions. When I am at work and the job I am doing just seems like a task I will never finish, or when it is late at night and I just can't sleep and my mind is cycling over and over, my safe place calms me every time.

Your safe place is yours alone and it is meant to relax you when you feel that you need to take yourself out of a bad situation. Your safe place is there for you always and it is up to you to determine when and how you use it.

Here is an example of how I used my safe place on a run, taken from my novel Why I Run.

Thought record:

On my Run this morning.

I am so proud of myself today and I am not afraid to show it. I am happy and proud. This morning on my run I spent my time in my safe place.

Moods:

Relaxed 100%, happy 100%

Sit:

I went to my safe place. My safe place is a tree. I imagined that I was a tall tree planted in my parents' back yard. My father's Ginkgo tree he planted when I was just six years old. I breathed deeply, inhaling through my leaves and exhaling through my roots. I just relaxed and did this for quite a while. Just thinking about what it must be like to be a tree. Not to have any expectations or worries, to have nothing to do but grow and grow, because I am a tree and that's what trees do.

I picture my father as a strong, young man planting me with his strong and caring, gentle hands. They are the same strong hands that held me as a baby and rocked me to sleep. They rocked my six older brothers as well. I think about how my father would water me after work and just stand there watching everyday as I grew.

As this tree I also watch a family grow around me never wanting to interfere or pass judgment or criticize, wanting only to breathe deeply and grow nice and slow, and watch this family grow as well. I watch soccer games. I watch this strong man build tree houses for his sons. I watch him play baseball with them and even build a pool and ice rinks for hockey games.

All along, my branches just grew and grew. I got taller and taller, children turned to teens and teens turned to men. The man who was once so strong also got older and older, and became a grandfather.

As a tree time, must be a very peaceful thing. As a tree, I just watch life flow by, with no obligations and no commitments. I just grow and learn just like I am doing in real life, growing and learning how to be myself. I love my safe place and I love who I am.

This was a goal I had made ever since I started therapy and found my safe place, which was not an easy task at the time. Now I am proud of myself, which is something I really haven't been able to say ever. I am proud because I did this. I reached a meditative state went to my safe place ran 8km in my safe place my tree. I am proud of myself because I have this safe place I can go to. I am worth changing and I am not afraid to be myself.

Enjoy your safe place.

Applying What You Have Learned

CHANGE YOUR NEGATIVE THINKING

Although this writing course may have seemed like a lot of work, the benefits from it are great on so many levels. Just learning that writing can be a wonderful way to express yourself and free yourself from the emotions you are feeling. Being able to just write them out on paper and get what you feel out of your mind and out into the open is huge accomplishment. Learning that our negative emotions are nothing to be afraid of or ashamed of is very important.

We all have times in our lives where we feel these emotions and learning to accept that is a big step. The power of writing is a gift that we all have and that we all can enjoy. The wonderful thing about it is that you are free to write what you'd like and feel what you want to feel. There is no right or wrong answer. Being able to see and read what you have written allows you to notice the way you are feeling, and shines a light on the negative thoughts you have. Being able to take that next step to change the way you think about yourself, your life and the people who are in it was the goal of this section.

Now that you have all these tools, you are now free to use them as you like. Make them your own and to apply them in your own ways to really grow as an emotionally aware person!

Applying these tools is actually a very fun exercise because now you have learned that writing is one of your best friends! Applying this is very easy, every morning write how you feel. Do you feel good? Write about why you feel good. Are you excited about your day? Write about it! Are you nervous, anxious, sad...? Write about it.

Before you go to bed, write about the good things that happened in your day. There are always good things that happen in your day, and you will now be able to see them because of the work have done over the last 5 weeks learning to apply the tools from this program!

USING WRITING AS A THERAPEUTIC TOOL

The tools we learned to apply when writing and practicing over and over again can be life changing. Learning to prove our negative thoughts wrong and in doing so being completely honest about what was bothering you (then changing it to a positive) is such a great feeling.

Learning that you always have these tools as a safety net in your life is both inspiring and rewarding. Using affirmations and saying them and writing them and believing them is a soul building activity. You now have an outlet you never had before, and you now have a place where you can sit and just let the power of your mind work in ways that you never thought were possible.

You are changing who you are and how you look at the world, and it feels good and exciting! Therapy doesn't have to be a dirty word. It can be a great experience where you learn to free yourself and inspire yourself and treat yourself with love and kindness. Using writing as therapeutic tool feels good!

MINDFULNESS AND GUIDED MEDITATION

We took creative writing and turned in it something completely different; we went from using it to change our way of thinking and free ourselves from our negative thoughts to helping us deal with our challenges which had happened in our lives. We then unlocked the power of our minds and learned how to slow down and enjoy life.

Learning how to practice mindfulness and applying it to guided meditation is proof of just how powerful the mind truly is. Plus, we learned that each and everyone one of us is capable of doing these great things and the only thing that separates us from others is the amount of practice that is put into the things we wish to accomplish in our daily lives. Learning mindfulness and guided meditation is proof of that! Being able to meditate and create beautiful places in our minds that you can taste, touch, smell, see and hear is proof that we can take our mind power and use it for wonderful things in our life.

Use mindfulness everyday. Practice it as often as you like and treat yourself with love, enjoying the small things in life. Guided meditation is a treat and you can now come up with so many different places in your mind. Use your overactive mind for you and no one else!

CREATE A SPACE PLACE

We used mindfulness and guided meditation and took it to the next level! We created a safe place for ourselves, a place we can go to in our minds and call our own. A place that is unique to each and every one of us! This safe place is your own personal place where you can go anytime to feel good about yourself and to also regroup and centre yourself whenever you feel the need to. We all deserve to be happy!

Your safe place is a major accomplishment, celebrate it, use it when you like to. Going to your safe place can only take five minutes. The key to putting it into practice is realizing how fast and easy it is to go there. Sometimes at work when a stressful situation occurs, I will just shut down and stop what I am doing to put off reacting in an emotional way and find a quiet place. The bathroom, I close my office door, I walk out side and lean against the wall. I get myself out of the stress physically so I can then do it mentally. I take five minutes and go to my safe place and I go there 100% ,the outside world can wait.

When I leave my safe place I take the power with me. The calm, the happiness, the strength, the wisdom of being able to first recognize when a situation happens in my life and then how different I feel after I use my safe place. Having your own safe place means you have tapped into the power of your mind and you are controlling your life and your emotions. It is a very special place! A very safe place. Take the time everyday to go to it and enjoy it and know just how powerful you are for having it.

FINAL EXERCISE

We will end this creative writing course like we started. You will now write freely about how this class has impacted your life and what your feelings are, and remember to write with great honesty and love using all the detail you would like. You have learned a lot. When you are finished writing out this exercise I want you to go back to the first page of your journal. Read what you wrote on the first day of starting this class and notice just how far you have actually come since then! Compare your thoughts and see just how much you have changed.

I hope that writing has helped you like it has helped me in my life. Make writing your best friend and embrace the true freedom of being able to write honestly and with love for yourself. Apply the tools we learned, and practice over and over again; let writing be a part of your everyday life.

Darcy Patrick

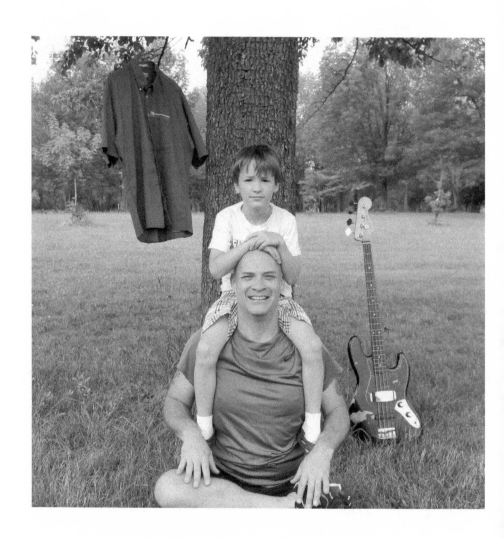

CPSIA information can be obtained
at www.ICGtesting.com
Printed in the USA
LVHW02s0735291217
561158LV00001B/16/P